Exercises for Being Mindfully: Volume Eight

Mindfulness Practices for Persons with Parkinson's Disease

9/3/2014
Parkinsons Recovery
Robert Rodgers PhD

Exercises for Being Mindfully
Mindfulness Practices for Persons with Parkinson's Disease
Volume Eight

Contents

The Parkinsons Recovery Mindfulness Series

Realistically speaking, how can the intense level of stress that aggravates the symptoms of Parkinson's disease be calmed? Better yet, how can they be quieted? My research over the past decade reveals that using your mind to drop the stress level down a notch or two always backfires. When you tell yourself:

- *Settle down!*
- *Take it easy!*
- *Stop being so stressed out!*

The stress level ratchets up, not down. Attempts to force the stress and anxiety levels to adjust downward induce an internally generated stress. They pile more stress on top of an excess of stress that already exists. There are certainly a sufficient number of external generators of stress in every one's life. Why infuse more stress that you create yourself, even with the best of intentions?

If the mind is not a useful technique to reduce stress, what is? The most eloquent answer I have for you is to become more mindful of what is experienced in the present moment. Becoming more mindful shifts you into the experience of the "now" which in itself is less stressful (unless you have been kidnapped by terrorists!).

It is stressful to anticipate events you imagine will occur in the future. The events we imagine rarely happen. Does this ring true for you? We all create unnecessary stress in our lives by how and where we focus our thoughts and attention.

It is stressful to agonize over the past. When we think about the past, we are much more likely to think about unpleasant experiences that induce stress. The past event itself was traumatic enough. Yet, we insist on reliving the trauma over and over again through our memories. It seems some of us just can't get enough stress in our lives.

The problem with upping the ante on stress levels is that – as you well know – symptoms of Parkinson's disease become worse. When you are not as stressed, your symptoms are far less problematic.

I have reached one solid conclusion from my ten years of research on Parkinson's disease. Symptoms will drive you crazy when you are stressed and are far less problematic when stress is under control.

Now, if you can't use your mind to become more mindful (which creates added stress in itself) how in the world can you quiet down a frantic lifestyle? I have concluded that the simplest and most effective solution to reducing stress levels is to become more mindful.

The transformation is possible step by step through these simple exercises you can do anywhere, anytime of the day. The Parkinsons Recovery mindfulness exercises are designed to focus your attention on the present moment as attention on either the past or the future is diverted. A renewed focus on the present moment reduces stress levels. Mindfulness is a lifestyle that will reduce stresses in your life if you set the intention to take a mindfulness practice seriously.

I recommend that you practice each of the exercises for a week or longer. Incorporate each practice into your regular routines and habits. Attempts to do all of the exercises simultaneously will likely induce more stress which – obviously – is contrary to the intent of a successful mindfulness program.

Give each exercise a little time and space. Invite the stresses in your life to dissipate. Allow the experience of each practice to engulf you. In so doing, watch the stresses in your life dip down to new lows along with a concurrent relief of any and all symptoms that you have currently been experiencing.

This volume is one out of nine I have developed to support the recovery of persons who currently experience neurological symptoms. A full listing of the Parkinsons Recovery Mindfulness themes follows:

Exercises for Being Mindfully
Mindfulness Practices for Persons with Parkinson's Disease
Volume Eight

Volume 1: Exercises for Seeing Mindfully

Volume 2: Exercises for Hearing Mindfully

Volume 3: Exercises for Noticing Mindfully

Volume 4: Exercises for Doing Mindfully

Volume 5: Exercises for Eating Mindfully

Volume 6: Exercises for Thinking Mindfully

Volume 7: Exercises for Feeling Mindfully

Volume 8: Exercises for Being Mindfully

Volume 9: Exercises for Intending Mindfully

Robert Rodgers, PhD

Parkinsons Recovery

www.parkinsonsrecovery.me

Olympia, Washington

Exercises for Being Mindfully
Mindfulness Practices for Persons with Parkinson's Disease
Volume Eight

How to be Mindful of the Present Moment

I have a challenge for you this week that I have been practicing now for some time. My own experience has been profound. Each and every encounter that you have with another individual, whether it is -

- *Over the phone*
- *Through an email exchange*
- *During a chat on the internet*
- *In person*

Think to yourself -

> *"There is a possibly this person may not be alive tomorrow."*

Let me be perfectly clear here. You are certainly not wishing that the person will die. Rather, you are honoring the reality that life is very fragile and very temporary. I have never met a person who is 140 years old.

You and I well know that we have friends and acquaintances who were alive and perfectly healthy one day. The following day they died from an entirely unexpected turn of events; automobile accidents, traumas, unexpected illnesses. It happens.

It happens to those who are one-day-old. It happens to those who are 100-years-old. Death comes to all living entities; animals, humans, everyone. We do not know when death will be knocking at our own door, but we can be assured it will pay us a visit eventually.

Recognizing this possibility enriches each and every encounter we have with another person. How many of you have experienced the following thought sequence? A family member or a treasured friend dies unexpectedly. You are very saddened. You are grieving. Some of your thoughts take the following form.

> *"The last time I saw my friend was three weeks ago. There were so many things I wish I had told them. I didn't really have time for them then because I was rushing off to another appointment. They wanted to hang out but I didn't have the time the last time I saw them alive. Oh how I wish I had had an opportunity once again to have that encounter. I would do it differently."*

I have had thoughts just like that in my life. Thoughts of regret and guilt will not surface when we are present and mindful of the present moment. The realization that it is possible (though of course not probable) that our friends and family may not be alive tomorrow is the thought that provides a powerful incentive to live in the present rather than being preoccupied with popping off to the next appointment.

The acknowledgment that every living being dies eventually enriches the practice of becoming mindful during each and every encounter. It enriches the loveliness of being alive in a body.

To summarize, with each and every encounter - whether it comes through email correspondence, a telephone conversation or face-to-face encounters – think the following:

> *"This person may not be alive tomorrow. We can never really know what the future has in store for anyone."*

Then, initiate the interaction. Notice how you feel about the exchange which ensues. Speaking for myself, all of my encounters became richer and more meaningful.

Why is that? I am not anticipating the future. Rather, I am living in the present moment, mindful that whatever thoughts I have and whatever feelings I may experience need to be expressed now. There may be no tomorrow to say what I had thought about saying yesterday but did not have enough time.

Deeper Meaning Behind Being Mindful of the Present Moment

I have learned an important lesson over the last several years. Denial runs deep in our veins. For some reason we are clearly able to see issues that other people have but are unable to acknowledge those same issues in ourselves. We insist on perceiving the world through our own distorted lens. It does not matter a hill of beans what the reality of the situation is.

So, there is no question about it. We deny – and I'm holding my hand up here – that life is very fragile indeed. I think to myself,

> *"I've got many years to live. I'm in a strong body. I'm healthy. I'm good to go for years and years."*

The truth of the matter is that this is a form of denial. There are bacterial infections out there that I may be exposed to and unable to release. There are delicate balances of potassium and magnesium in my body that must be maintained for life to be sustained. These could spin out of balance anytime.

There are certain systems in our body that maintain the sleep cycle. It could be that when driving I will slip off to sleep and veer off the road. Who knows what might happen tomorrow?

9

I'm not intending to be pessimistic or dire in any sense of the word. What I'm really doing with this mindfulness challenge is to respect the magical mystery of each and every moment. When we do just that, each moment is enriched immeasurably.

We can all continue to have conversations with others when we are only partially present. When we choose to switch the habit of listening partially and haphazardly to being fully and completely present, we become fully engaged with the present moment. We connect to the other person with our heart and soul.

When we part, we know that we have made a profound encounter and connection. The experience of being present in the moment taps into the juice of our life force. It feeds our energy and enthusiasm for life

The Japanese have a very special tradition. When a person leaves, whether through walking or through a car or through a train or plane, the person waving them goodbye waits until the car or the plane or the person has disappeared. Why? This may be the last time they will ever see that individual. It is a divine ritual for all of us to adopt whether we are Japanese or not!

The chant quoted below is taken from a Zen monastery of Jan Bays, who is a medical doctor and author of **How to Train a Wild Elephant.** I invite you to say it every day this week.

"May I respectfully remind you that life and death are of supreme importance.

Time swiftly passes by and opportunity is lost.

When this day is past, our days of life will be decreased by one.

Each of you should strive to awaken.

Awaken! Take heed. Do not squander our life."

Phones

Most people live very busy, active lives. We turn from one task to the next without any pauses. Thoughts cycle from one to the next without interruption. We operate on a continuous fast forward rush of activity without ever stopping until our heads hit the pillow at the end of the evening.

My mindfulness challenge this week offers you an opportunity to slow the quick pace of life down. Remember. This quick pace is a key factor that induces stress in your life. As you well know, stress is a sure bet to make symptoms much worse. The idea here is to reduce the level of stress in your life. It needs to become manageable for your symptoms to reverse.

How can you slow the quick pace of your life down with the mindfulness challenge this week? It is actually easy to do. The challenge is this. Each time the telephone rings – whether it is a land line or a cell phone – instead of immediately rushing to pick up the receiver and say,

"Hello. Robert here, how can I help you?"

Pause. Take three slow, mindful breaths after the phone rings the first time. The phone of course will ring three, four, five, maybe even six times as you pause from what

12

you were doing to what you are about to do. Once your three breaths are completed, pause. Center yourself. Pick up the receiver and say slowly and mindfully -

"Hello. Robert here. How may I help you, today?"

Obviously substitute your name for mine when you answer. We do not want to proliferate the world with more Roberts.

There is a huge difference in the degree of stress that is created according to how we engage a simple task like answering the telephone. When we rush to answer, the stress level jumps. When we answer mindfully, the stress level dips. The conversation starts from a more comfortable place energetically. The person on the other end of the line also does not feel rushed or stressed. When they do, our own stress level will rise along with the neurological symptoms.

Becoming more mindful when we answer the phone also nurtures our own sanity. It helps to maintain that critical balance in our body. It enables our neurological system to flourish and function precisely the way it was designed to function in the first place.

Have fun each time the telephone rings. Remember, change the your habit of answering the phone by doing the following when the phone does ring:

© Parkinsons Recovery

1. *Take three, long, slow, mindful breaths.*
2. *Pause at the end of those three breaths.*
3. *Center yourself as you prepare for a new experience.*

Be excited about what the person on the other end of a line will want to discuss with you. Reduce stress in your life by using this very simple but powerful mindfulness exercise.

When we slow ourselves down, we treasure each moment rather than rushing off to the next one. When we are in a rush to get to the next moment, we miss that one too because by then, we are busy rushing off once again. Without any pauses, we miss the rich experience of every I moment.

Give yourself a regular dose of pauses every day. I think pauses give you better results than any prescription medicines you might be taking to suppress symptoms.

Deeper Meaning Behind Pausing Before Answering Your Phone

Have you enjoyed the pause that refreshes? Have you been pausing and taking three breaths before answering your phone when it rings, whether it is a cell phone or a land line? Have you been taking those three delicious slow breaths? Have you been pausing? Have you been centering yourself before answering? If so...

- *Has your degree of impatience reduced over the last several days?*
- *How about the anxiety that you consistently feel here and there or continuously?*
- *Are you less irritated?*

I hope so! If you continue this mindfulness practice, chances are good that the degree of impatience, anxiety and irritation in your life will be soothed and quieted. Now, that in itself is a huge benefit from simply changing the habit of how you answer the phone, eh?

First of all, many people actually are not aware and do not realize that they are constantly impatient, anxious and irritated, all of which are high octane fuel for stress. Permit me offer an example of what I have noticed about myself.

As I am falling asleep, I have made it a practice to assess the muscular tension in my body. The result of these evening assessments has been shocking. Muscles in my face are always tensed up around my mouth, neck and eyes. With my intention, I can release and reduce that tension before I fall asleep. I never really knew I held so much tension in my body, especially my face.

I suspect that many people are not aware that they too are constantly and continuously anxious. They too hold tension throughout their body: in their muscles, legs, arms, neck, face and even their scalp. If the physical body is always in a continuous state of tension, it is not going to have any opportunity to come back into balance. Only a body that is in balance can settle down an overactive neurological system.

There is an advantage to the fact that phones tend to ring randomly. The invitation to pause when the phone rings will afford an opportunity to access and acknowledge the degree of irritation, anxiousness and impatience you may currently be experiencing. Once recognized, it becomes possible to sooth that anxiousness, impatience and irritation so that you are better able to be present in the moment. You cannot succeed in calming anxiety if you do not even acknowledge it!

There is a second, more profound implication for this mindfulness challenge. When there happens to occur an irritating and troubling exchange with another person who you just talked with on the phone, it is normal to carry that irritation into the next encounter or even the remaining encounters for the rest of the day.

How many times have you decided you wanted to talk with someone else, perhaps a boss, perhaps a co-worker, perhaps a family member or spouse and, as you approached them, they had a sour look on their face? Something is obviously troubling them. Do you have an opportunity to talk about what you wanted to talk with them about? The answer typically is "no way." They are going to be preoccupied with what has just happened to them whether it was earlier in the day or, as is often the case, what happened days and days prior to your encounter with them. It is often a wise decision to walk away and hope for a better time to have a conversation when a person is in a state of turmoil and distress.

We carry these irritating encounters from one encounter to the next. The stress accumulates in the tissues of our body. Eventually we become a continuously anxious person. Everything seems to set us off. We are not able to release that irritation because we cannot seem to unload and release it. It literally sticks to our backs like super glue.

It is magical to realize that each encounter with another person can be a fresh, interesting experience. When we treat each encounter as such, the experience becomes much more positive and life-giving rather than negative and life draining. If we engage any encounter with a sour attitude because the last person that we talked with put us in a very bad mood, every encounter that we have for the remaining day, for tomorrow, for the week, for the month and perhaps even for the rest of our lives is typically going to be pretty sour too.

This is why there is a benefit to pausing each time the phone rings. By pausing, we have the opportunity to clear out all of the irritation and anxiety that has accumulated up to that point in the day for whatever reason. By pausing we are able to dump out the anxiety that has built up during the day and make a fresh start with each new encounter.

I must say I have truly relished doing this particular assignment. I am oftentimes deep into doing some type of writing or work on my computer when the phone rings. My response is oftentimes irritation,

> *"I'm almost done with my task and here somebody wants to talk with me. Give me a break. I only need a couple of more minutes. Can't they wait?"*

So, there the irritation is. It is intense. If I carry that irritation into how I answer the phone, the person on the other end of the line is going to immediately sense my mood:

> *"Oh my goodness, this is not a good idea to talk with Robert right now. I should only take a couple of seconds of his time."*

18

What a big difference it can make if I pause between those the two tasks. After taking several breaths, it becomes obvious there will be plenty of time to complete the task that I was working on prior to the call. I can always finish my work after the conversation. I can center myself. I can then be ready to engage the conversation with the individual who is calling with a new attitude, an attitude that does not carry with it the baggage of impatience, anxiety, irritation and stress that has accumulated during the day.

I hope this particular mindfulness challenge will be useful to you in identifying anxiety that may have been lingering in your physical body not only during the day but throughout your entire life. If your experience is anything like mine, you have likely been unable to acknowledge, recognize and honor the tension that is held throughout the tissues of your body.

May this mindfulness challenge be an opportunity to stop, re-group and have marvelous exchanges with each and every person that you encounter from this day henceforth. May the technique also be useful for reducing the tension that lingers throughout all the tissues of your body.

Slow It Down

The mindfulness challenge this week is to slow everything down. Yes, this will take more time to accomplish the same tasks but the benefits are significant. Slowing each and every task down will have a profound impact on reducing your stress level. Try it. You will like it.

What do I mean when I say, "Slow it down?"

- *If you are chopping up red peppers for a dinner, when I say "slow it down" I mean chop up those red peppers slowly and mindfully.*
- *If you are walking from the kitchen to the living room, when I say "slow it down" I mean to take each step one by one with mindful consciousness, planting one foot after the other using conscious intention.*

Slow down each and every task that you initiate this week – whatever the task entails – from opening up a car door and getting in, to simply going to the telephone and picking it up to answer a call (as you have already been practicing!).

Many individuals who confront neurological challenges have a tendency to push up against any and all tasks. This persistent forcing and pushing fertilizes stress in the body. Because the nature of neurological challenges means that

20

you must somehow slow down activities, a war is declared against the enemy of getting tasks done efficiently and effortlessly. If we cannot get a task done in a timely fashion, a response familiar to most people is to push through it regardless of the consequence.

"No pain. No gain."

Yes, tasks can be completed quickly and successfully when you push through them, but the cost is high. Stress levels sore. Symptoms flare.

There is a heavily researched theory in the management literature known as goal setting. When you set high, hard goals, you achieve more and produce more. The theory is well proven. What are the long term consequences? Stress levels sore. Symptoms flare. The executive is praised for reaching their goals, but they have to quit their jobs at an early age because of a heart attack.

Reverse the tendency to rush through tasks. End the battle to set high goals and accomplish them quickly. These behaviors only make symptoms worse. Goal setting behavior is just the food your body needs to produce stress hormones. As you well know now, high stress levels create troublesome neurological problems.

Slow down each and every activity. Enjoy and relish what it means to open up the door to your car, what it means to walk from the kitchen to the living room, what it means to actually cut a red pepper.

To succeed with the challenge to slow down you must plan ahead. Give yourself at least twice if not three times as much time to accomplish each task. If you are a person who always makes a list of tasks that must be accomplished each day, cut in half the number of items on your list. Give yourself plenty of time to accomplish each and every task during the day.

Notice the profound impact slowing down has on your stress level. Notice what happens to your symptoms. You are sure to notice a welcome difference! Celebrate the miracle of what it means to be mindful with what you do and how you do it, moment to moment.

Deeper Meaning Behind Slowing It Down

Where did my mindfulness challenge of the week to "slow it down" actually originate? On the Parkinsons Recovery cruise to Alaska there was a most delightful woman who told her own story of recovery. She was in her 80s and showed little evidence of Parkinson's symptoms. It was clear by her own report that she had experienced Parkinson's symptoms for more than two decades. It was also clear that she had been able to manage her life quite beautifully.

During a time when the entire group was together we were all sharing stories about what therapies and approaches helped people reverse their symptoms. This very wise woman reported that what had been most helpful to her was to plan ahead. When she planned ahead she could give herself plenty of time to do each and every task without stressing out.

> *"For example, if my husband and I have decided that we're going to have a dinner party, I don't wait until the last minute to begin preparing for the party. I begin preparing the day before. The day of the party I start quite early in the morning preparing everything that needs to be ready by the time of the party with regard to the food and cleaning up the house. By starting early I mindfully*

23

attend to each and every task that needs to be completed before our guests arrive.

"Twenty years ago", she continued, "I would have waited until just a few hours before the party started and rushed to get everything ready. Now, because that creates so much stress and it aggravates my symptoms so desperately, I have learned a different way of living. I mindfully attend to each and every task. I'm centered. I'm clear. I'm able to focus on the task of the moment rather than worrying about whether everything will actually be done, finished and ready when my guests arrive."

That is how she approached all tasks in her life; slowly and mindfully, not just tasks involving preparations for parties. She always gave herself the gift of having plenty of time to finish each and every task during the day.

If our day is packed with too many commitments, the difficulty (as it turns out) is that with each activity, we are always watching the clock. We are always thinking,

"I must complete the task at hand quickly, because the next task has to start in 15 minutes."

Or we think,

"I promised my friend that I would be at the coffee shop at ten o'clock. I must complete this baking

*task before I actually see her because I promised
her that I would bring her my special brownies for
her birthday."*

Et cetera. Et cetera. In other words, we are always
focused on the future. We are always anticipating that we
must complete what we are doing now in order to be on
time or have enough time to do what we have decided we
must do by the end of the day. We are forever rushing
from one task to the next without being mindfully
attentive to any task at hand. We are not living in the
present. We are always anticipating the future.

Slow it down. Reduce the number of tasks that you expect
to complete in any given day. Marvel at the reduction in
stress that your body will experience.

I can assure you that your body will thank you profusely. I
also predict that your symptoms will dissolve like a dirty
snowball in the springtime. May you have a delightful
time as you slowly execute each and every task that you
undertake.

Impatience

The invitation this week is to be totally mindful of your thoughts regarding getting something done quickly. Become aware in the moment of any and all situations when you become impatient; when you want to get whatever you are doing in the moment over with quickly.

For example, when you are driving, notice if there are situations when you think to yourself or even say out loud:

> *"Can't that driver ahead of me go a little faster?"*

Or, consider situations where you are waiting for a friend to return a phone call or return an email. You find yourself thinking over and over again,

> *"Why doesn't he return my call? Why doesn't he return my email? I'm ready to hear from him now not in five minutes from now."*

Or, perhaps you are out in the yard doing a little yard work. Your thoughts are,

> *"I can't wait for this task and this chore to be done so I can do the fourth chore on my list. I will never be done with all my chores if I don't finish this one in 10 minutes."*

After recognizing the intensity of your impatience I have another suggestion for you. Each time during the day when you acknowledge, recognize and observe there is a situation where you are being impatient – when you want something to get over quickly for whatever reason – I have a very simple two-word question that I'd like to suggest you ask yourself:

"Then what?"

In other words, when I am done doing what I am doing right now, when I have finished this task ask,

"Then what?"

Enjoy the invitation this week to observe any and all situations when you find that you have become impatient. I have been doing this task myself all week and am surprised by how many times I find myself being terribly impatient. I would have told you last week that I am a very patient person, but this week? I don't think so.

Deeper Meaning Behind Impatience

What is the deeper meaning behind situations where we find that we are impatient with what is happening, whatever the situation might entail? There is a good chance that underneath impatience is an unstated belief. That belief is:

> *"There is not enough time. There is not enough time in the day for me to do what it is that I need to do and that I want to do."*

This is a belief that is not true and has never been true. There is plenty of time to do whatever it is that we set our intention to do. If we think that there is not enough time - if that is the belief that we hold near and dear to our hearts - then guess what?   There will never be enough time to do what it is that we would like to do and want to do.

There is a companion issue associated with being impatient. If you are impatient with a particular task or with doing many tasks throughout the day, it is often the case that we think to ourselves,

> *"I'm ready to be done with this task because I have something much more fun and much more interesting that I want to do right now. I don't*

want to run out of time so that I can't enjoy the
task I really want to do."

For example, as you are washing the dishes after dinner you find yourself rushing through this task. Why? There is a video that you are craving to watch. You have been thinking about watching this video all day long. You want to get the dishes finished quickly because you want to be sure you have enough time to watch that exciting video. The thought is,

"Washing dishes really isn't very much fun."

In other words, you are not present to the chore of washing dishes.

The reality is that everything we do can be a fascinating experience even if we have done the very same task 12,150 times (which would be the task of washing the dishes for most of us!). Each task is an occasion to have a new experience. If the task involves - as in my example - washing the dishes, then,

- *Feeling the water over our hands.*
- *Feeling the texture of the soap.*
- *Watching the dishes change as the soiling clears.*
- *Placing the dishes in the dish drain as they form a unique mosaic.*
- *Listening to the sounds that surround us as we wash the dishes.*

- *Smelling the dish soap.*
- *Watching the bubbles.*
- *Feeling the texture of being present in the moment as we feel our clothes nestle against skin.*

Enjoying each and every moment of this experience means that each time we wash the dishes it winds up being a totally new experience. We can be endlessly interested and fascinated with a task as routine as washing the dishes.

There are no experiences that are boring in and of themselves. We only make them so with our beliefs and thoughts. We impose a static label of boredom on certain tasks that is arbitrary and unfounded.

If we rush to finish a task because we are eager to begin another, we are living in the future. We are projecting out onto something that has not yet happened. When you finally do get to the next task, it oftentimes does not meet our fantasies about how interesting, pleasurable and engaging it will be. And then of course we begin anticipating the next experience long before the present task is finished.

If we actually reflect back on any activity that we had declared to be routine and boring – something we have to do because it has to be done by someone – chances are we might actually recognize that the activity can be

© Parkinsons Recovery

interesting. We were not aware of what we were doing because we were not being mindful.

It is easy to be impatient when chronic symptoms present themselves; impatient that they vanish, impatient that those symptoms resolve quickly. When we are in the moment, the rattletrap of untrue beliefs and thoughts suddenly vanishes. We occupy our thoughts, our emotions and our feelings to what it is that we are experiencing in the present moment.

Hopefully you have now been observant of situations when you have been impatient over the past several days. Have you found that you are impatient more frequently than you had acknowledged previously (as was my case)? What was your answer to the question:

> *"Now when I get through with this task, what next?"*

How many times did you find yourself asking the question,

> *"What next?"*

You know and I know that the ultimate final answer to that question is death. Are you really rushing as fast as you can to that end state of death? Is that what this is all about?

1. *Slow down!*
2. *Be present in the moment.*

I can assure you that as you monitor the degree to which you find you are impatient, you will be able to more mindfully be present to each and every moment. Stress will be reduced. When stress is reduced, symptoms will dissolve like a snowball in the summertime.

Transitions

The mindfulness challenge this week is admittedly onerous
and difficult. If you choose to accept the challenge, I must
warn you in advance that you will indeed find it to be
perplexing and frustrating. You will likely find that you
repeatedly forget to actually do what I am about to
suggest.

The focus of the mindfulness exercise this week is on
transitions as you move from one space to another. We
face continuous transitions throughout each day. Because
most of us do often anticipate the future, we miss the
experience of the actual transition moment. We anticipate
what we are about to encounter in a room we are about to
enter rather than fully and completely experiencing the
transition from one space to the next.

The challenge is the following. For each closed door that
you confront throughout the week, stop before you open
the door. Take a breath in and out. Then, open the door
and enter the new space. You may well encounter as
many as two hundred closed doors in a single day that
need to be opened. You may well forget to stop, take a
breath and then open the door for half, three-fourths or
who knows, all of the doors that you encounter in any
given day.

33

Please accept this invitation as a fun challenge anyway.
Each and every door that you encounter that is closed,

1. Stop.
2. Take a slow breath in - then out.
3. Open the door.
4. Enter the new space mindfully.

Have fun with the onerous and difficult challenge of the week as you begin the most rewarding of all challenges to become present in each and every moment of your life. May you have a magnificent week opening and closing the doors of your life.

Deeper Meaning Behind Transitions

There is no doubt about it. Our bodies are in continuous states of transition. One day we wake up and have a mild headache. The next day we wake up and have a pain in our left leg. The third day we wake up and there is no pain, but there is a surge of energy that is running throughout our entire body.

Transitions happen continuously throughout each day. Every second of our lives there is a ticker tape of messages that are being transmitted by our body to our mind.

What is the interpretation of all of this? Suppose there is a change to what is happening in your body. A symptom has surfaced that has never been experienced previously. What is your typical response?

Most people make an immediate jump to the future. There is an instant transition from the "room" (or body) we have been living in to the next "room" (or a body with different symptoms) without any thought about what it means to enter into the new "room" (or the different body so to speak).

There is an interpretation that is typical for individuals who have a diagnosis of a chronic condition like Parkinson's. The typical interpretation follows a familiar pattern:

> *"Oh my goodness, something else is going wrong with my body. I can't believe it. Don't I have enough symptoms as it is? What's wrong now? What therapy am I going to have to go get now? Geez."*

And so on and so forth... In other words, we immediately skip to the future without stopping to experience the underlying meaning of what is happening to us and our body in the moment. In so doing, we do not receive or understand the message that our body is trying to send to us.

The changes in the body are surely, as you can well appreciate, not all bad. Many of them are positive, meaningful and useful transitions that the body is making toward a state of health and wellness.

With many therapies, you will actually feel worse before you begin feeling better. When meridians are opened up - when surges of energy begin running through our body - it will very likely feel different and even strangely unfamiliar.

Yet, when the interpretation is

"What is wrong now?"

Rather than pondering ...

"Hello. What is here now"?"

We miss being present to the experience. We instantly draw the false conclusion that we are getting bad news. Our body is often giving us signals that are rewarding and supportive of all the work that we are doing to become symptom-free. The body is always trying to help us recover and reverse symptoms so that we can lead full and productive lives.

The exercise of stopping before opening any door invites a focus on being present in the moment – of being present to any transition that is made from one state to the next. As I mentioned in the introduction to the exercise, we pass through many doors in any given day. Our body also makes many transitions throughout any single day – many more than the number of closed doors that we confront. Our bodies can potentially make more like 800 or 900 different transitions in a day as it rocks, shakes and rolls its way to recovery and wellness. The body is in a continuous state of transitions and change.

The invitation then is to continue the exercise to stop, take a breath and then - and only then - open up each door that you confront. When you confront obstacles – and here the obstacle is a door that is shut – consider an alternative interpretation. You face a temporary transition. Something has shifted. The invitation is to stop, to take a breath and to say:

> *"What's here now in my body? What wonderful message is my body conveying to me now?*
>
> 1. *I've stopped.*
> 2. *I've paused.*
> 3. *I've become mindful.*
>
> *I am listening now in the moment with no bother or worry about whatever implications this experience might have for me in a minute, or two minutes, or tomorrow or next year. It does not matter what awaits me in the next room.*

If you take this exercise seriously you will begin to appreciate the many different ways door knobs feel when you touch them. You will begin to appreciate how the new space feels to you when you enter it.

Enjoy the many transitions you will make over the coming days as you pass through one door after another. Enjoy the experience of stopping, taking a breath and then opening up the door that separates the two spaces. When you take mindful notice of the transition - each one will have a different feel to it just as your body will feel differently with each new transition. Each transition is unique. Each can be a precious experience.

By being mindful of all transitions, recognize and honor the difference in the spaces to be entered (when compared to the rooms that are left). When you enter new spaces may there be renewed interest and awareness about what is present. When your body enters into new states, may there be renewed interest and awareness about what is present too.

May you relish all transitions this week whether they consist of passing through doors or experiencing the continuous ebb and flow of symptoms.

Posture

The challenge and invitation this week is to become more mindful moment to moment of your posture. Do you really have a truthful picture of what your posture is really like? We all see ourselves from the front. And, from the front, we do not look too terribly bad no matter how twisted or contorted the posture. What about from the side? How do you really look from the side when someone else sees you from that angle?

Go to a mirror and in your natural way of standing, look at yourself from the side. What does your posture look like when you examine at yourself in a mirror from the side just as a doctor might do?

- *Are you humped over?*
- *Is your belly sticking out?*
- *Is your head lunged downward?*

What do your family members and your friends say about your posture? Ask them.

> *"Tell me about my posture. Is it good or am I slouching a bit these days?"*

Perhaps your immediate response is:

- *I don't need to look in the mirror.*
- *I don't need to ask my family members.*
- *I know my posture stinks.*

What thoughts have been rattling through your mind as you have been pondering this week's challenge? Have you been thinking thoughts like:

> *"Oh, I can't do anything about my posture. I'm too old. We all know that as people age, their posture always goes to pot."*

Challenge that belief. It is not true.

> *"There's no way I have strong enough muscles to do anything about my posture. You know, I have neurological challenges."*

This belief in itself is perfectly designed to ensure that you will be a hunchback permanently as you age.

Challenge all such beliefs. None of them are true. Anyone in any condition can improve their posture.

How is this accomplished? I do not belief the long term solution is to go to a single therapy session or training workshop. I believe posture is improved moment to

41

moment. As you sit, if you happen to watch the TV or if you happen to sit in front of your computer, be attentive. What is your posture like?

1. *Is your back straight?*
2. *Are your feet solidly planted onto the floor?*
3. *Are you sitting on the edge of your seat where it is possible for your posture to be improved?*

If not, why not for this week at any rate, sit on the edge of your chair when you eat? Many people have a habit of slouching when they eat. Challenge yourself with sitting upright as you bring each bite proudly up to your mouth?

Notice when you walk what your posture is like. Be attentive. How does your body feel? Are you feeling strain in certain muscles? Poke that chest out as you walk. Notice how your head will lurch not forward, but upward so that you walk proudly and confidently. Think to yourself as you walk: Chest forward.

Become attentive to your posture as you stand. Notice whether it feels as though more weight is being placed on one leg. If so, this habit will place undue pressure on your hips. When you even out the weight placed on the left and right legs and feet you will not need a hip replacement. Supplements or medicines will not be necessary to repair damage to your hip bones and muscles. Healthy hips are a function of good posture and frequent movement.

In summary, the mindfulness challenge this week is become more attentive to your posture when

1.   *Sitting*
2.   *Eating*
3.   *Walking*
4.   *Standing*

It is particularly useful to be attentive to your posture when you are standing – perhaps waiting in a line at the grocery store to check out. How are you standing at the pump as you wait for your gas tank to fill? Are you slouched? Shift the posture. See how you feel when you make the shift. It is amazing how a little shift in body weight to the right or left sides can help reduce many symptoms.

Needless to say it is not possible or practical to be mindful of your posture every single moment. That intensity of focus would not be very functional or useful. It would also create more stress. Allow this mindfulness exercise and challenge to unfold gently.

At a minimum, be mindful of your posture several times during the day. When you notice an imbalance, shift your posture to a more balanced position whether this means moving your chest forward or shifting your weight from one side to the other. Make a change at least one time a day. Your body will thank you.

Deeper Meaning Behind Being Attentive to Posture

When we become depressed about our health situation —
when our negative thought forms eat up our energy — our
body will show sure fire evidence that our life force is
being drained. Our energy level and physical presence
show what is really happening to us inside.

Transformation of thought forms can make a huge
difference. Transforming the following negative thought -

> *"There's no way I can feel better,"*

Into a positive thought,

> *"Of course anyone can recover if they set their
> intention to do so,"*

Is the difference that makes a huge difference to the pace
of recovery.

Transformation of negative thought forms into positive
ones can be very challenging. Negative thoughts start
spinning in our mental hamster wheel at the most
inopportune moments. There are two ways to shift the
negative thought patterns into positive ones.

We can choose to shift the thought patterns that are not
in our best and highest good and the physical

44

improvements will follow. Or, we can shift the physical aspects of our posture and quiet the hamster wheel of negative thinking.

Either of these approaches will succeed but for many people, it is far more difficult to transform the habits of negative thought patterns. Your invitation this week is to focus on transforming the physical aspects of poor posture.

- *If we are slumping down ...*
- *If we are hunching our backs ...*
- *If our head is tilted downward ...*
- *If we are always looking toward the ground ...*

We are in a posture of surrender. We are giving up. We are telling the world,

> *"Well, I've given it my best try and, you know what, I think it's time to give up."*

If you have decided that giving up is not an option for you, then accept my challenge this week to shift the aspects of your posture that do in fact signal surrender. Place your highest priority on transforming the aspects of your posture that are evidence of disease and illness. Stand up straight as possible. Carry a physical presence that communicates what you want truly and genuinely to manifest.

1. Hold your head up.
2. Posture your body proudly.
3. Straighten your spine.
4. Shift your chest forward.
5. Assume the gaze of unflinching confidence.

Assume the posture of an athlete. Assume the posture of a ballerina. Assume the posture of an individual who has all the confidence in the world to accomplish whatever they set their intention to accomplish.

Our posture is compelling evidence of what is going on internally. Shift the physical posture if it is out of balance and you also begin to transform what is happening internally. If at any moment during the day you notice a decrease of energy or a bit of depression slipping in, what do you do?

This week embrace the mindfulness practice of shifting your posture. Your breathing will improve. Your thought forms will transform instantly. Shift your posture and everything shifts.

Can you do it? Of course you can do it. Anyone can do it. Perhaps if you are having muscle challenges or weakness it will be difficult to have that perfect posture, but that is not the point here. The point is to shift your awareness consciously and mindfully, moment to moment. Muscles can and do get stronger even for those who are a century old.

You can see miracles happen by this one very simple mindfulness exercise. Good posture means you are solidly on the road to recover from any and all symptoms that you currently experience.

Have a magnificent time as your posture improves

Minute by Minute
  Hour by Hour
    Day by Day
      Week by Week

Transforming bad posture does not have to happen instantly. It happens gradually as you become aware of how you are holding and moving your body moment to moment. Chest out!

Have a magnificent and proud week. The exciting news is that when we are able to stand tall and proud, we manifest recovery quicker.

© Parkinsons Recovery

Parkinsons Recovery Programs

Has your work on these exercises been stress free? Has it been helpful in reducing your symptoms? I certainly hope so! This is the primary reason I developed the mindfulness exercises in the first place.

If you struggled with pacing out these mindfulness exercises so as not to induce more stress, there are several Parkinsons Recovery programs that might help expedite your recovery. My Parkinsons Recovery Mindfulness Program sends the mindfulness exercises in an email to you each and every week. The initial exercise is sent to your email address on day one of the week and the deeper implications are sent four days later. The Parkinsons Recovery Mindfulness Program takes one full year to complete as each exercise is introduced one week at a time. For more information visit:

www.stress.parkinsonsrecovery.com

Parkinsons Recovery Memberships involve a variety of support websites that are essential to recovery. A difference mindfulness exercise is posted each week. For more information on Parkinsons Recovery memberships visit:

www.parkinsonsrecovery.org

Of course, the approach that works for many people is to purchase a single volume of the Parkinsons Recovery Mindfulness program at a time as you have already done! See the introduction for a listing of all nine Parkinsons Recovery Mindfulness volumes.

Thank you for Your Support

On behalf of the thousands of followers of Parkinsons Recovery, I want to thank you for your purchase of this booklet. One hundred percent (100%) of the profits purchases of my books and programs help subsidize the many free services I offer through Parkinsons Recovery -

www.parkinsonsrecovery.com

For information about other products, services and programs visit -

www.parkinsonsrecovery.me

www.ingramcontent.com/pod-product-compliance
Lightning Source LLC
Chambersburg PA
CBHW070501290526
45790CB00003B/1047